The Ultimate Keto Bread Recipes for Beginners

Super-Tasty Recipe Collection of Keto Bread to Enjoy your Weight Loss Journey and Look Beautiful

Jessica Simpson

© **Copyright 2020 - All rights reserved.**

The content contained within this book may not be reproduced, duplicated or transmitted without direct written permission from the author or the publisher.

Under no circumstances will any blame or legal responsibility be held against the publisher, or author, for any damages, reparation, or monetary loss due to the information contained within this book. Either directly or indirectly.

Legal Notice:

This book is copyright protected. This book is only for personal use. You cannot amend, distribute, sell, use, quote or paraphrase any part, or the content within this book, without the consent of the author or publisher.

Disclaimer Notice:

Please note the information contained within this document is for educational and entertainment purposes only. All effort has been executed to present accurate, up to date, and reliable, complete information. No warranties of any kind are declared or implied. Readers acknowledge that the author is not engaging in the rendering of legal, financial, medical or professional advice. The content within this book has been derived from various sources. Please consult a licensed professional before attempting any techniques outlined in this book.

By reading this document, the reader agrees that under no circumstances is the author responsible for any losses, direct or indirect, which are incurred as a result of the use of information contained within this document, including, but not limited to, — errors, omissions, or inaccuracies.

Contents

Turmeric Cauliflower Bread 10

Chewy Poppyseed Bread 13

Buttery Skillet Flatbread 15

Spiced Focaccia Bread 17

Cauliflower Tartar Bread 19

Keto Bagel Loaves 21

Pumpkin Bread 24

Keto Pumpkin Bread 26

Cashew Bread 28

Blueberry Bread 30

Garlic & Herb Focaccia 33

Lemon & Rosemary Shortbread 35

Pistachio And Cocoa Squares 39

Keto Chocolate Bombs 41

Lemon Fat Bombs 43

Cocoa Balls 44

Peanut Butter Fat Bombs 46

Raspberry Cream Fat Bombs 48

Almond Butter Cinnamon Bars 49

Pina Colada Fat Bombs 51

Red Velvet Fat Bombs 52

Walnut Brownie Balls 54

Raspberry Cheesecake Balls 56

Mocha Truffles 58

Vanilla Cheesecake Fat Bombs 59

Salted Macadamia Keto Bombs 60

Peppermint And Chocolate Keto Squares	62
Ginger Patties	64
Coconut Truffles	65
Keto Ramekin Bread	67
Apple Cider Bread	68
Keto Cream Cheese Bread	70
Low Carb Flax Bread	72
Gluten-free Garlic Bread	75
Zucchini Bread With Walnuts	77
Cheesy Keto Garlic Bread	79
Morning Hamburger Loaves	81
Savory Sage Bread	83
Cinnamon Bread	85
Cloud Bread	87
Almond Flour Bread With Olive	89
Low Carb Blueberry Bread	91
Jalapeno Cornbread Loaves	93
Walnut Bread	95
Sweet Potato Bread	98
Coconut Bread	100
Flax Seed Bread	101
Keto Breadsticks	103
Cranberry Bread	105

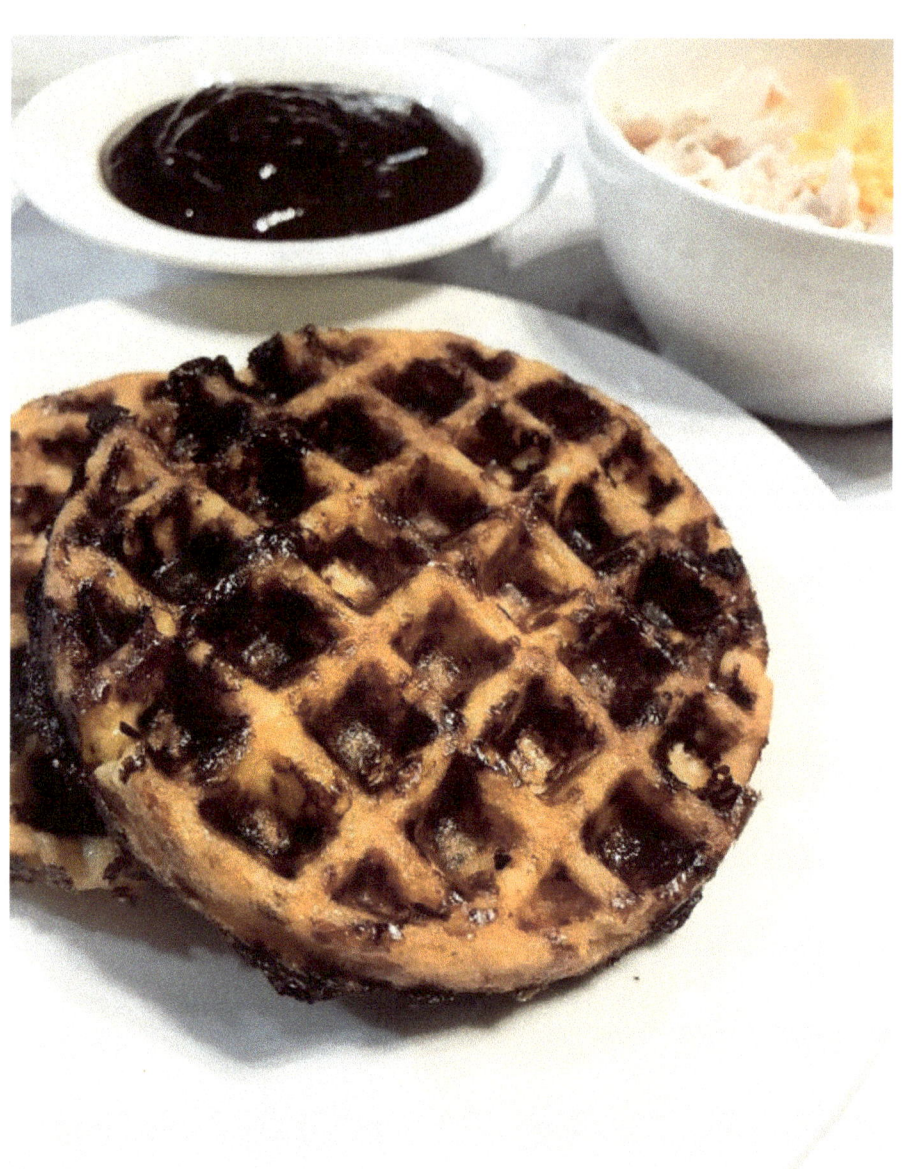

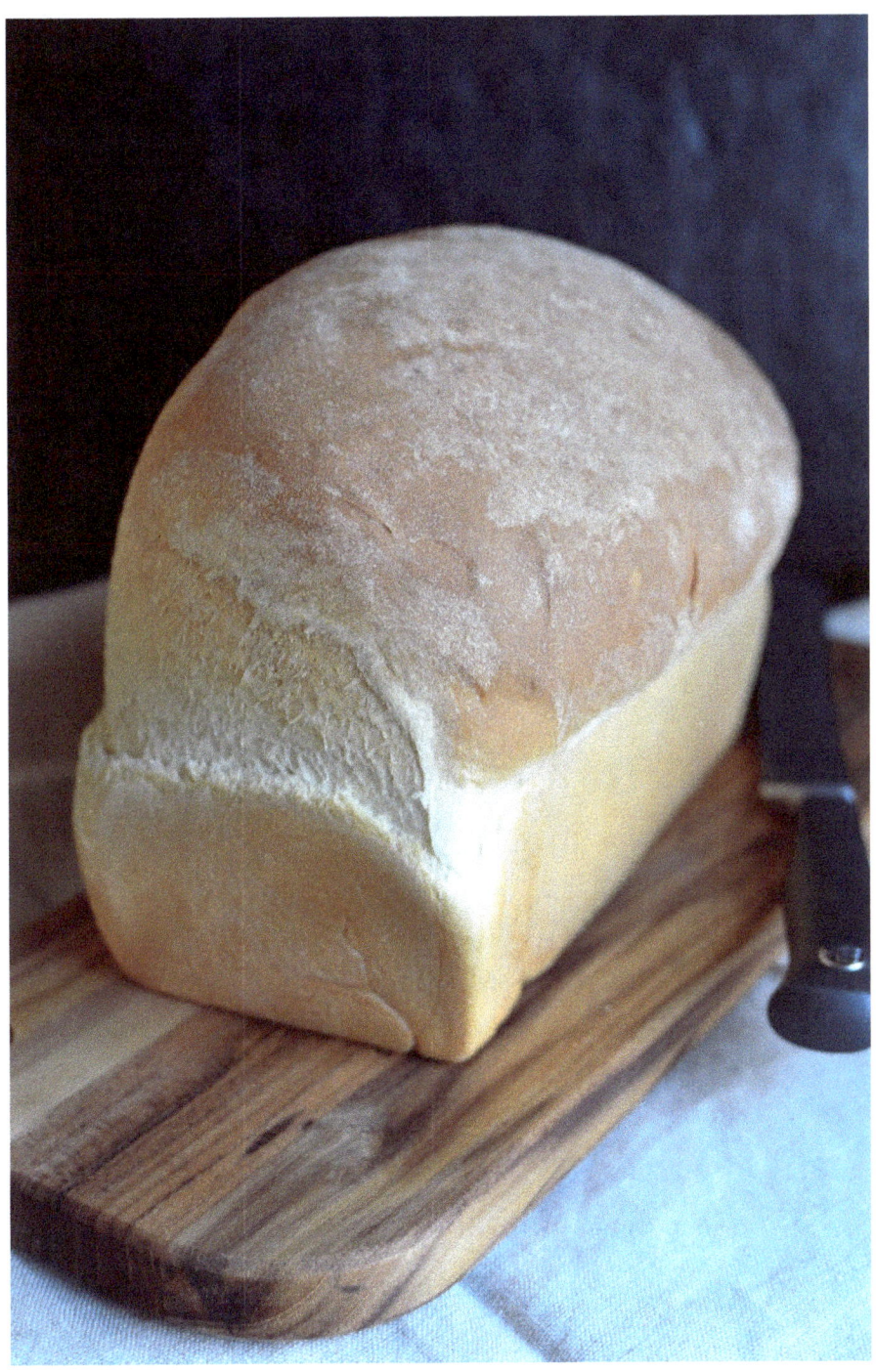

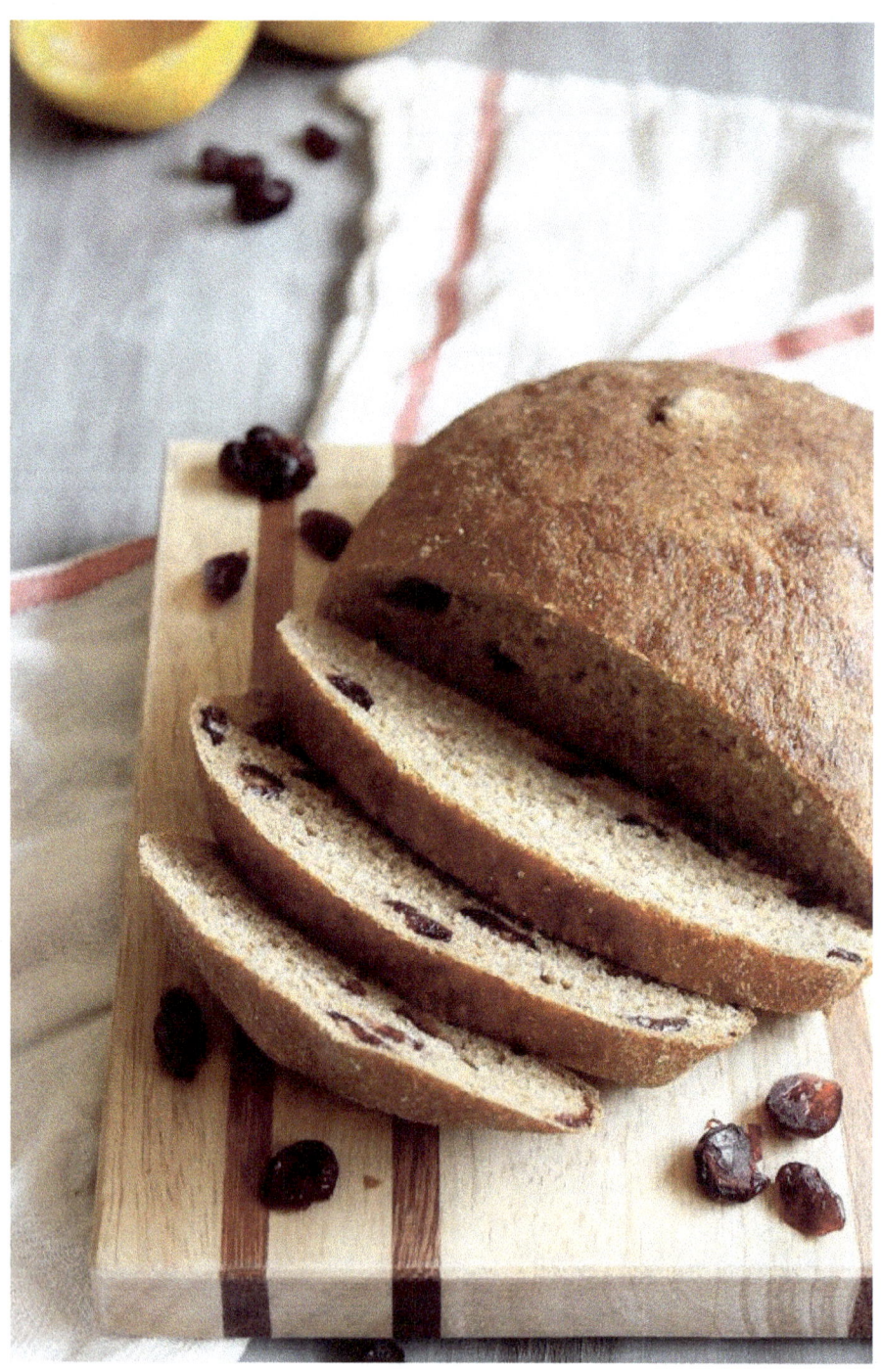

Turmeric Cauliflower Bread

Servings: 6

Cooking Time: 30 Minutes

Ingredients:

- 2 cups cauliflower rice
- 2 eggs
- 2 tbsp coconut flour
- ¼ tsp ground turmeric
- Pinch each of salt and pepper

Directions:

1. Preheat your oven to 400 degrees F. Layer a baking sheet with wax paper.
2. Add a teaspoon of water to the cauliflower rice in a microwave safe bowl.
3. Cook for minutes on High.
4. Transfer the cauliflower rice to a kitchen towel and squeeze out excess water.
5. Mix drained cauliflower rice with coconut flour, eggs, salt, black pepper, and turmeric in a bowl.
6. Make equal-sized rounds out of this mixture and place them in a baking sheet.
7. Bake them for 30 minutes until golden brown.
8. Serve.

Nutrition Info: Calories 113 Total Fat 8.4 g Saturated Fat 12.1 g Cholesterol 27 mg Sodium 3mg Total Carbs 9.2 g Sugar 3.1 g Fiber 4.6 g Protein 8.1 g

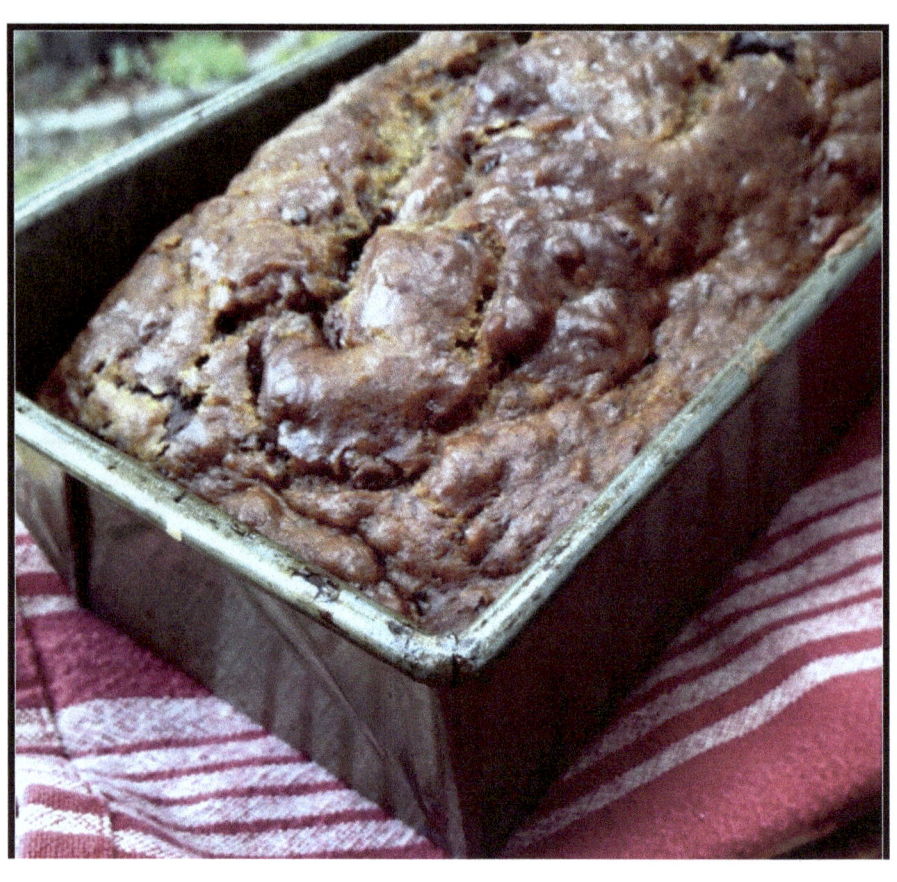

Chewy Poppyseed Bread

Servings: 8

Cooking Time: 20 Minutes

Ingredients:
- ½ cup coconut flour
- 2 tsp baking powder
- ¾ tsp xanthan gum
- 12 oz pre-shredded mozzarella
- 2 large eggs
- Topping
- 1 tsp sesame seeds
- 1 tsp poppyseed
- 1 tsp dried, minced onion
- ½ tsp coarse salt
- 1 tbsp butter melted

Directions:
1. Preheat your oven to 350 degrees F. Layer a loaf pan with a silicone liner.
2. In a bowl, combine baking powder, coconut flour, and xanthan gum and set it aside.
3. Add cheese to a microwave safe bowl and melt it for seconds in the microwave.
4. Stir in eggs and flour mixture then mix well to form a smooth dough.

5. Spread this dough in a greased loaf pan.
6. Whisk sesame seeds with salt, dried onion, melted butter, and poppyseeds in a shallow dish.
7. Brush the poppyseed mixture over the bread.
8. Bake it for 20 minutes until golden brown.
9. Serve fresh.

Nutrition Info: Calories 251 Total Fat 24.5 g Saturated Fat 14.7 g Cholesterol 165 mg Sodium 142 mg Total Carbs 4.3 g Sugar 0.5 g Fiber 1 g Protein 5.9 g

Buttery Skillet Flatbread

Servings: 4

Cooking Time: 10 Minutes

Ingredients:

- 1 cup almond flour
- 2 tbsp coconut flour
- 2 tsp xanthan gum
- ½ tsp baking powder
- ½ tsp salt
- 1 whole egg + 1 egg white
- 1 tbsp water (if needed)
- 1 tbsp oil, for frying
- 1 tbsp melted butter, for brushing

Directions:

1. Mix xanthan gum with flours, salt, and baking powder in a suitable bowl.
2. Beat egg and egg white in a separate bowl then stir in the flour mixture.
3. Mix well until smooth. Add a tablespoon of water if the dough is too thick.
4. Divide the dough into equal portions and then spread them into ¼-inch thick rounds.
5. Place a large skillet over medium heat and heat oil.

6. Add one round in the skillet and cook for 1 minute per side.
7. Cook the remaining rounds in the skillet and place them in a platter when done.
8. Mix butter with salt and parsley.
9. Brush butter over the bread and enjoy.

Nutrition Info: Calories 272 Total Fat 18 g Saturated Fat 5 g Cholesterol 6.1 mg Sodium 3 mg Total Carbs 4 g Fiber 3 g Sugar 4 g Protein 0.4 g

Spiced Focaccia Bread

Servings: 9

Cooking Time: 25 Minutes

Ingredients:

- 1 cup almond flour
- 1 cup flaxseed meal
- 7 large eggs
- ¼ cup olive oil
- 1 ½ tbsp baking powder
- 2 tsp minced garlic
- 1 tsp salt
- 1 tsp rosemary
- 1 tsp red chili flakes

Directions:

1. Preheat your oven to 350 degrees F.
2. Whisk almond flour with flaxseed meal, spices, and baking powder in a bowl.
3. Stir in garlic, eggs, and olive oil and beat this mixture well until smooth.
4. Grease a 9x9-inch baking pan with cooking spray.
5. Pour the prepared batter in the baking pan then bake for 2minutes.
6. Allow to cool for 10 minutes then slice.
7. Serve.

Nutrition Info: Calories 245 Total Fat 19.9 g Saturated Fat 4.g Cholesterol 32 mg Sodium 597 mg Total Carbs 3.4 g Sugar 1.9 g Fiber 0.6 g Protein 10.29 g

Cauliflower Tartar Bread

Servings: 6

Cooking Time: 50 Minutes

Ingredients:

- 3 cup cauliflower rice
- 10 large eggs, yolks and egg whites separated
- ¼ tsp cream of tartar
- 1 ¼ cup coconut flour
- 1 ½ tbsp gluten-free baking powder
- 1 tsp sea salt
- 6 tbsp butter
- 6 cloves garlic, minced
- 1 tbsp fresh rosemary, chopped
- 1 tbsp fresh parsley, chopped

Directions:

1. Preheat your oven to 350 degrees F. Layer a 9x5-inch pan with wax paper.
2. Place the cauliflower rice in a suitable bowl and then cover it with plastic wrap.
3. Heat it for 4 minutes in the microwave. Heat more if the cauliflower isn't soft enough.
4. Place the cauliflower rice in a kitchen towel and squeeze it to drain excess water.
5. Transfer drained cauliflower rice to a food processor.

6. Add coconut flour, sea salt, baking powder, butter, egg yolks, and garlic. Blend until crumbly.
7. Beat egg whites with cream of tartar in a bowl until foamy.
8. Add the egg whites mixture to the cauliflower mixture and stir well with a spatula.
9. Fold in rosemary and parsley.
10. Spread this batter in the prepared baking pan evenly.
11. Bake it for 50 minutes until golden then allow it to cool.
12. Slice and serve.

Nutrition Info: Calories 104 Total Fat 8.9 g Saturated Fat 4.5 g Cholesterol 57 mg Sodium 340 mg Total Carbs 4.7 g Fiber 1.2 g Sugar 1.3 g Protein 3.3g

Keto Bagel Loaves

Servings: 4

Cooking Time: 25 Minutes

Ingredients:

- 1 cup almond flour
- ¼ cup coconut flour
- 1 tbsp psyllium husk powder
- 1 tsp baking powder
- 1 tsp garlic powder
- Pinch salt
- 2 medium eggs
- 2 tsp white wine vinegar
- 2 ½ tbsp ghee, melted
- 1 tbsp olive oil
- 1 tsp sesame seeds

Directions:

1. Preheat your oven to 320 degrees F.
2. Whisk garlic powder with almond flour, coconut flour, baking powder, salt, and psyllium husk powder in a suitable bowl.
3. Beat eggs with vinegar in a separate bowl then stir in ghee slowly while still whisking.
4. Add dry flour mixture and mix well until smooth then let the dough rest for 3 minutes.

5. Slice the dough into 4 equal pieces then spread them into thick rounds.
6. Place them onto a baking sheet layered with parchment paper.
7. Cut a small hole in the center of each round using a cookie cutter.
8. Sprinkle sesame seeds on top then bake for 25 minutes.
9. Enjoy.

Nutrition Info: Calories 220 Total Fat 20.1 g Saturated Fat 7.4 g Cholesterol 132 mg Sodium 157 mg Total Carbs 63 g Sugar 0.4 g Fiber 2.4 g Protein 6.1 g

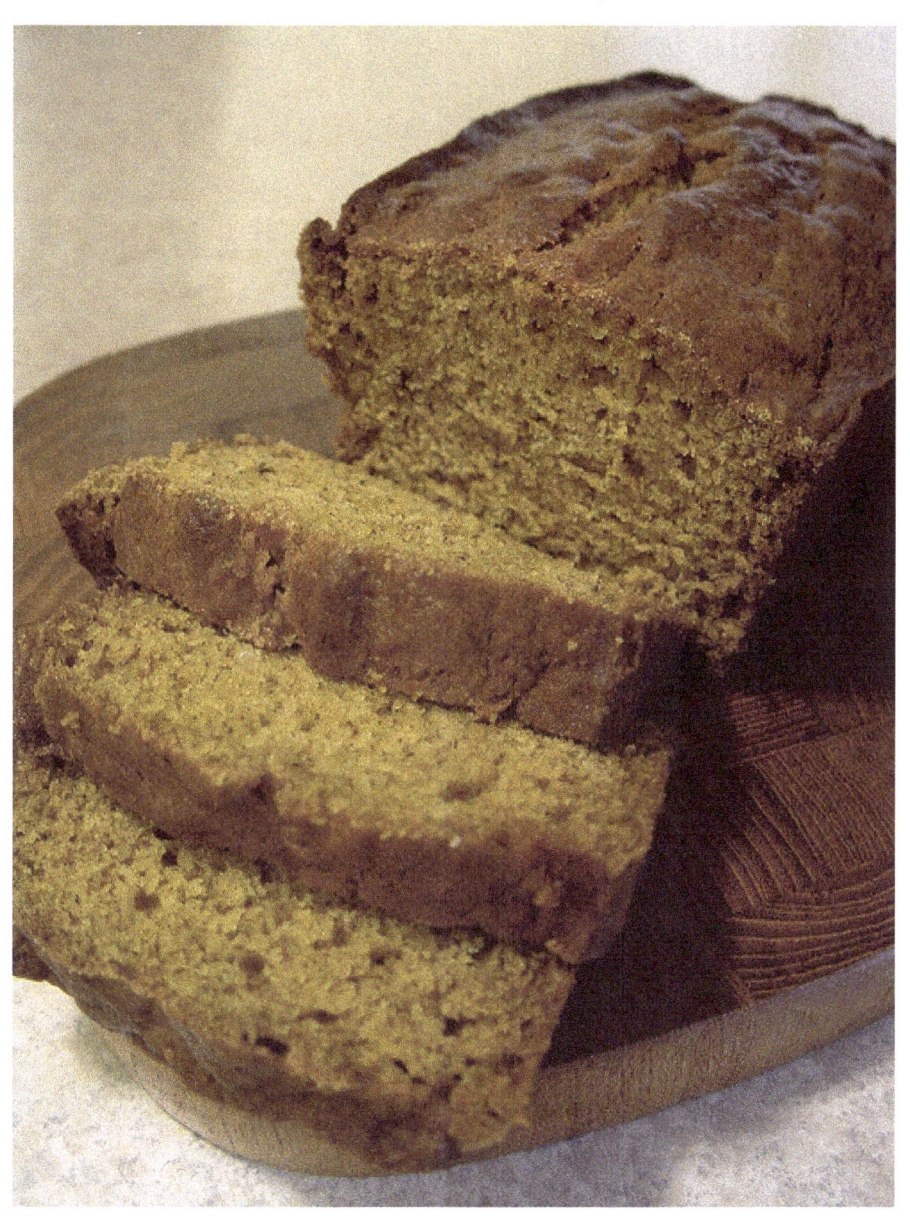

Pumpkin Bread

Servings: 5

Cooking Time: 65 Minutes

Ingredients:

- ¾ Cup of almond flour
- 2 to 3 egg whites
- 4 Tbsps of pumpkin puree
- 4 Tbsps of almond milk
- 2 Tbsps of Psyllium Husk powder
- 1Teaspoon of baking powder
- 1 Teaspoon of pumpkin spice
- ¼ Teaspoon of salt

Directions:

1. Preheat your oven to 345 F and then line a medium sized loaf pan with parchment paper.
2. Put a medium pan into the rack of your oven and pour water in that pan.
3. Combine your dry ingredients all together in a deep bowl and mix very well until it is perfectly incorporated.
4. Add the egg whites and the pumpkin puree to your dry mixture.
5. Pour the almond milk into the mixture and knead it until you form solid dough.

6. Knead the dough until it becomes dough smooth to the touch and place your dough into the loaf pan you have prepared.
7. Bake the pumpkin loaf in the Bain-marie for around 60 to 65 minutes.
8. When a toothpick you insert comes out clean, turn off the heat and remove your loaf pan from the oven.
9. Let the loaf bread rest for 15 minutes.
10. Slice and serve.
11. Enjoy your bread!

Nutrition Info: Calories: 75;Fat: 4 g;Carbohydrates 2.5g;Fiber: 0.7 g;Protein: 3 g

Keto Pumpkin Bread

Servings: 10

Cooking Time: 55 Minutes

Ingredients:

- ½ cup butter, softened
- 2/3 cup erythritol sweetener
- 4 large eggs
- ¾ cup pumpkin puree, canned
- 1 tsp vanilla extract
- 1 ½ cup almond flour
- ½ cup coconut flour
- 4 tsp baking powder
- 1 tsp cinnamon
- ½ tsp nutmeg
- ¼ tsp ginger
- 1/8 tsp cloves
- ½ tsp salt

Directions:

1. Preheat your oven to 350 degrees F and grease a 9x5-inch piece of wax paper and fit into a loaf pan.
2. Beat butter with sweetener in a mixer until foamy.
3. Whisk in eggs one by one while continuously beating the mixture.
4. Stir in vanilla and pumpkin puree then mix again.

5. Take a separate bowl and mix almond flour with other dry ingredients in this bowl.
6. Stir in wet eggs mixture and combine them well.
7. Pour this batter evenly into the prepared loaf pan.
8. Bake the bread for 55 minutes until it is done.
9. Allow it to cool on a wire rack then slice to serve.

Nutrition Info: Calories 165 Total Fat 14 g Saturated Fat 7 g Cholesterol 632 mg Sodium 497 mg Total Carbs 6 g Fiber 3 g Sugar 1 g Protein 5 g

Cashew Bread

Servings: 6

Cooking Time: 50 Minutes

Ingredients:

- 2Tbsp of vegetable oil to grease your loaf pan
- 2 and ½ cups of whole raw cashews
- 7 Tbsp of coconut flour
- 8 Beaten large eggs
- ½ Cup of milk
- 4 Teaspoons of apple cider vinegar
- 4 teaspoons of baking powder
- 1 Teaspoon of salt

Directions:

1. Put a heatproof dish with around 2 inches of water and place it into the bottom rack of the oven and then preheat it to around 325 F.
2. Grease the loaf pan you are going to use and then line the pan with the parchment paper and press it to the bottom.
3. Set the dish aside and meanwhile, put all together the coconut flour, the cashews, the eggs, the milk, the apple cider vinegar, the salt and the baking powder and process the mixture for around to 40 seconds.

4. Once the mixture becomes very thick, add 1 to 2 tbsp of water and process again until the mixture becomes smooth.
5. Transfer your batter to your already prepared loaf pan and bake it in the oven for minutes.
6. Once the bread gets a brown color, remove it from the oven and discard it from the parchment paper.
7. Slice the bread; serve and enjoy it!

Nutrition Info: Calories: 1;Fat: 13 g;Carbohydrates: 4.6g;Fiber: 2 g;Protein: 7 g

Blueberry Bread

Servings: 6

Cooking Time: 25 Minutes

Ingredients:

- ½ Cup of cashew butter
- ¼ Cup of ghee, coconut oil or butter
- ½ Cup of almond flour
- ½ Teaspoon of salt
- 2 Teaspoons of baking powder
- ½ Cup of unsweetened almond milk
- 6 Beaten eggs
- ½ Cup of frozen wild blueberries

Directions:

1. Preheat your oven to around 350 F.
2. In a deep and large bowl, mix the cashew butter and the butter for around 30 seconds; then stir very well.
3. In a separate large bowl; combine the almond flour with the salt and the baking powder; then pour the cashew butter and keep whisking.
4. Mix the almond milk and the eggs; then pour it into the bowl and whisk.
5. Break your frozen blueberries and then gently stir it into your batter.

6. Line a medium loaf pan with a parchment paper and then lightly grease it with spray.
7. Pour the batter into your medium loaf pan and bake it for around 45 minutes.
8. Set the bread aside to cool for 20 minutes.
9. Slice the bread and toast it; then serve and enjoy it!

Nutrition Info: Calories: 160;Fat: 12.8 g;Carbohydrates: 5.7g;Fiber: 1.1g;Protein: 6.9 g

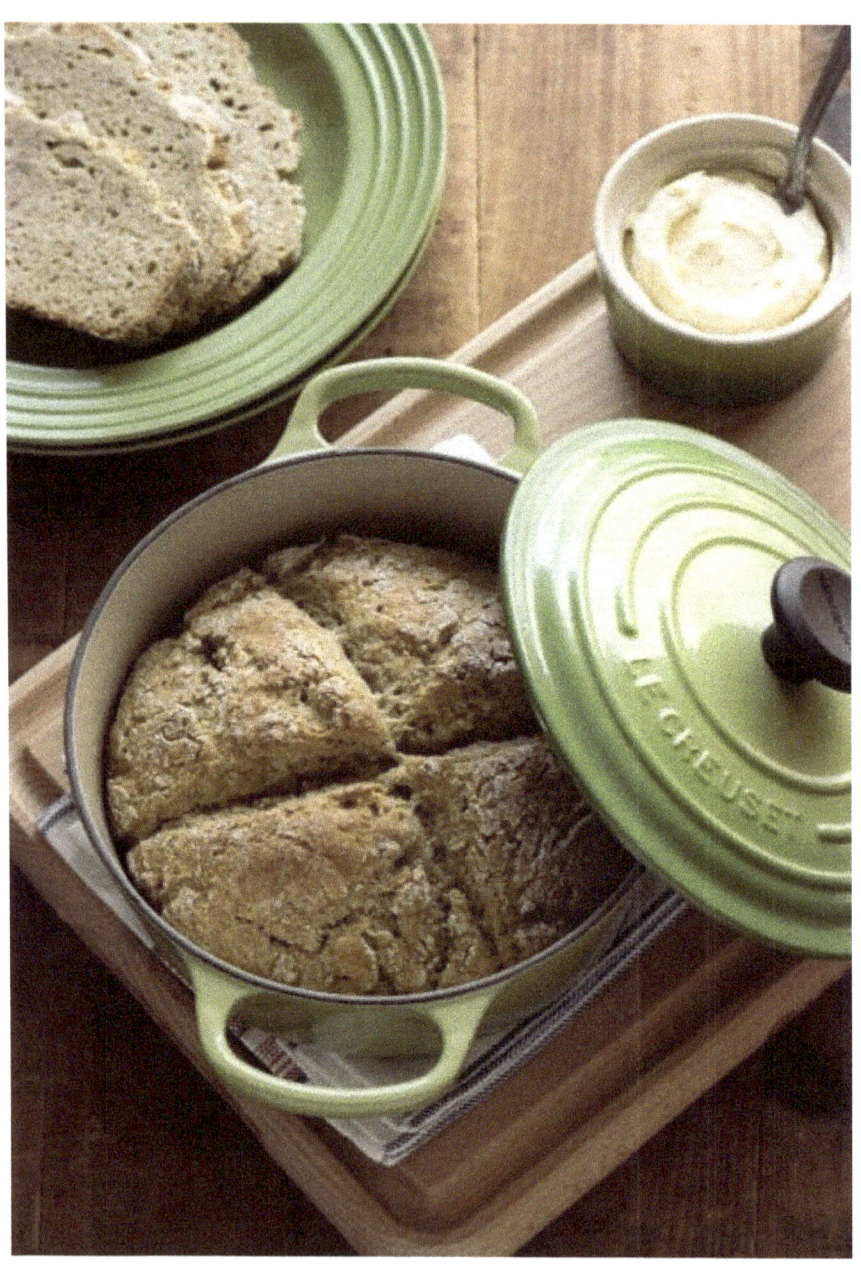

Garlic & Herb Focaccia

Servings: 8

Cooking Time: 20 Minutes

Ingredients:

- Dry Ingredients
- 1 cup almond flour
- ¼ cup coconut flour
- ½ tsp xanthan gum
- 1 tsp garlic powder
- 1 tsp flaky salt
- ½ tsp baking soda
- ½ tsp baking powder
- Italian seasonings, to garnish
- Salt flakes, to garnish
- Wet Ingredients
- 2 eggs
- 1 tbsp lemon juice
- 2 tsp olive oil + 2 tbsp olive oil to drizzle

Directions:

1. Preheat your oven to 350 degrees F. Layer an 8-inch baking pan with wax paper.
2. Whisk the dry ingredients in one bowl then beat the egg with oil and lemon juice in another.
3. Mix these two together in a large bowl until smooth.

4. Spread this dough in the prepared pan evenly.
5. Bake the bread for 10 minutes then drizzle olive oil over it.
6. Continue baking for another 10 minutes until brown.
7. Sprinkle salt and Italian seasoning over it.
8. Enjoy.

Nutrition Info: Calories 121 Total Fat 12.2 g Saturated Fat 2.4 g Cholesterol 110 mg Sodium 276 mg Total Carbs 3 g Fiber 0.g Sugar 1.4 g Protein 1.8 g

Lemon & Rosemary Shortbread

Servings: 10

Cooking Time: 15 Minutes

Ingredients:

- 6 tbsp butter
- 2 cups almond flour
- 1/3 cup granulated Swerve
- 1 tbsp freshly grated lemon zest
- 4 tsp fresh squeezed lemon juice
- 1 tsp vanilla extract
- 2 tsp rosemary
- ½ tsp baking soda
- ½ tsp baking powder

Directions:

1. Mix 2 cups of the flour with baking soda and baking powder in a large bowl.
2. Stir in Swerve and mix well then add the lemon zest and lemon juice.
3. Add butter and vanilla to a bowl and heat it in the microwave for seconds on high.
4. Mix well then pour it into the flour mixture along with rosemary.
5. Whisk well until smooth then knead it into a long log.

6. Wrap the dough in plastic wrap. Refrigerate for 30 minutes.
7. Meanwhile, let your oven preheat at 350 degrees F.
8. Remove the wrap and slice the dough log into ½-inch thick slices.
9. Place the slices on a cookie sheet greased with butter.
10. Arrange the dough slices on the baking sheet then bake them for 15 minutes.
11. Let them cool for 10 minutes and serve.

Nutrition Info: Calories 267 Total Fat 24.5 g Saturated Fat 17.4 g Cholesterol 153 mg Sodium 217 mg Total Carbs 8.4 g Sugar 2.3 g Fiber 1.3 g Protein 3.1 g

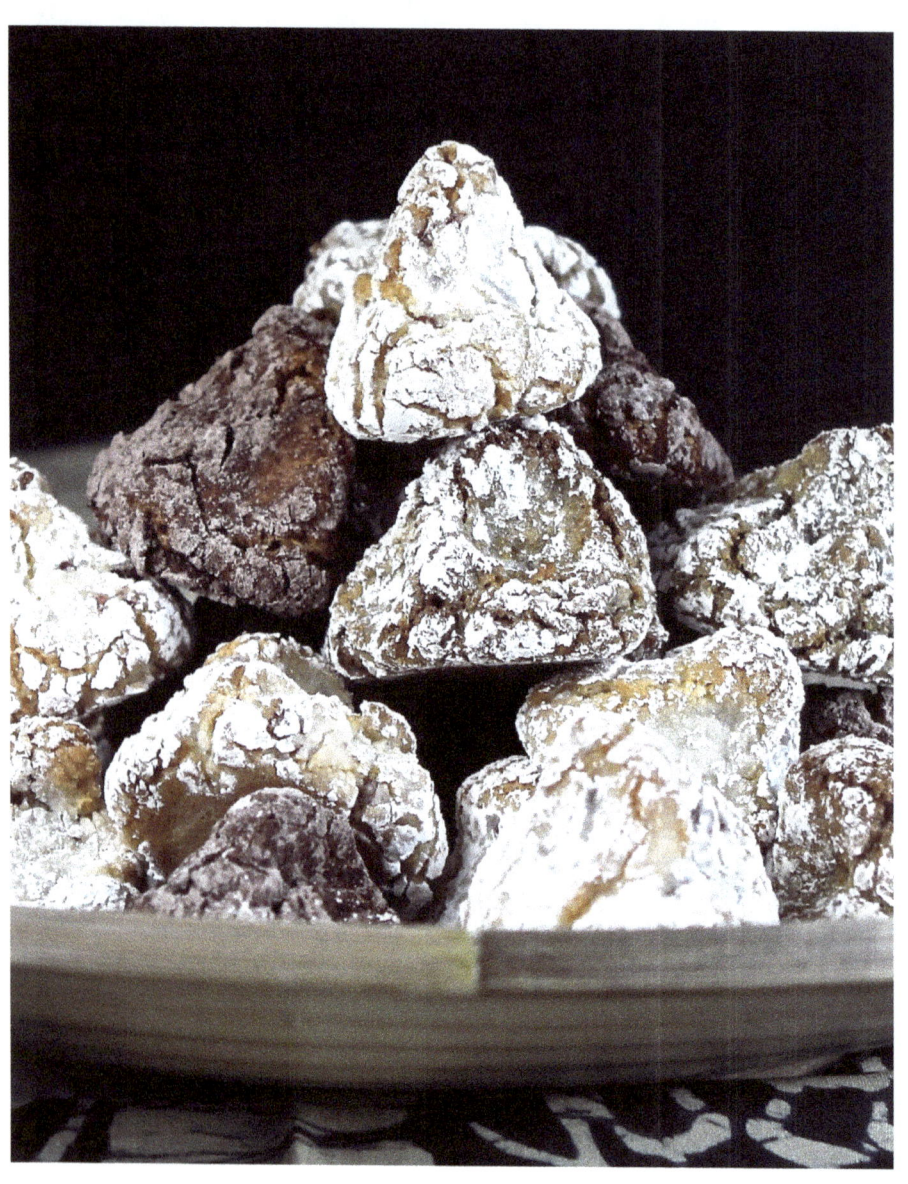

Pistachio And Cocoa Squares

Servings: 13

Cooking Time: 5 Minutes

Ingredients:

- ½ Cup of finely chopped and cacao butter
- 1 Cup of roasted almond butter
- 1 Cup of creamy coconut butter
- 1 Cup of firm coconut oil
- ½ Cup of full fat coconut milk, chilled for an overnight
- ¼ Cup of ghee
- 1 Tablespoon of pure vanilla extract
- 2 Teaspoons of chai spice
- ¼ Teaspoon of pure almond extract
- ¼ Teaspoon of Himalayan salt
- ¼ Cup of chopped raw pistachios, shelled

Directions:

1. Grease a square baking pan of about 9" sand line it with a parchment paper; make sure to leave a little bit hanging on both sides to help you unmold easily; then set aside.
2. Melt the cacao butter in the oven for about 30 seconds and reserve it.
3. Add the roasted almonds, the coconut butter, the coconut oil, the coconut milk, the ghee, the vanilla

extract, the spice, the almond extract, the salt and the chopped pistachios to a large mixing bowl and mix very well starting with a low speed; then increase the speed and mix until the mixture become airy.
4. Pour the mixed and melted cacao butter into that of the almond and keep mixing on a high speed until you get an incorporated batter.
5. Transfer the prepared pan; then evenly spread the batter and sprinkle with the chopped pistachios.
6. Refrigerate your batter for about 4 hours or for an overnight.
7. Cut into about 36 squares; then serve and enjoy!

Nutrition Info: Calories: 170; Fat: 17 g;Carbohydrates: 3.1g;Fiber: 1.5g;Protein: 2.4 g

Keto Chocolate Bombs

Servings: 12

Cooking Time: 0 Minutes

Ingredients:

- 2 Cups of smooth peanut butter
- ¾ Cup coconut of flour
- ½ Cup of sticky sweetener
- 2 Cups of sugar-free chocolate chips

Directions:

1. Start by lining a large tray with a parchment paper and set it aside.
2. In a large mixing bowl, combine all your ingredients together except for the chocolate chips, and combine your ingredients very well until it is completely combined
3. If your batter is too thick or is crumbly, you may add a small quantity of milk or water
4. With both your hands, try forming small balls from the batter and arrange it over a the already prepared lined tray and freeze for about 10 minutes
5. While your peanut butter balls are in the freezer, melt the sugar-free chocolate chips in the microwave for about 30 seconds to about 1 minute

6. Remove the peanut butter from the freezer; then carefully and gently dip each of the balls into the melted chocolate
7. Repeat the same process until all the chocolate balls are covered in chocolate and arrange over a platter
8. Once you finish covering all the balls, place the balls in the refrigerator for about 20 minutes or just until the chocolate firms up
9. Serve and enjoy your delicious chocolate balls!

Nutrition Info: Calories: 95;Fat: 9.7 g;Carbohydrates: 2.4g;Fiber: 1.2g;Protein: 3 g

Lemon Fat Bombs

Servings: 15

Cooking Time: 10 Minutes

Ingredients:
- 9 oz full fat cream cheese
- 4 oz full fat ricotta cheese
- 3 Tbsp flaxseed oil
- ½ cup fresh lemon juice
- Zest of 2 lemons
- ¾ cup coconut flour
- 1 tsp Stevia/your preferred keto sweetener

Directions:
1. Line a baking tray with baking paper
2. Combine all ingredients until fully incorporated
3. Roll the mixture into 15 balls and place them onto your lined tray
4. Pop the tray into the fridge for an hour so the balls can set and firm up
5. Store the bombs in an airtight container in the fridge

Nutrition Info: Calories: 102; Fat: 8 grams; Protein: 3 grams; Total carbs: 4 grams; Net carbs: 2 grams

Cocoa Balls

Servings: 9

Cooking Time: 0 Minutes

Ingredients:

- 1 Cup of almond butter
- 1 Cup of coconut oil, at room temperature
- ½ Cup of unsweetened cocoa powder
- 1/3 Cup of coconut flour
- ¼ Teaspoon of powdered stevia
- 1/16 tsp of pink Himalayan salt

Directions:

1. In a small pot and over a medium high heat, melt the almond butter and combine it with the coconut oil.
2. Add the coconut flour, the cocoa powder and the Himalayan salt and stir.
3. Add the stevia and mix again; then let your mixture cool.
4. Pour the mixture in a large bowl and transfer it to the freezer to solidify for about 60 to 90 minutes.
5. Once solidified, remove the bowl from the freezer and form it into balls.
6. Form balls from the batter and arrange the balls over a tray lined with a parchment paper.
7. Refrigerate the balls for about 15 minutes.

8. Serve and enjoy your delicious Ketogenic bombs!

Nutrition Info: Calories: 157| Fat: 12.6 g;Carbohydrates: 3.4g;Fiber: 1.8g;Protein: 3.7 g

Peanut Butter Fat Bombs

Servings: 18

Cooking Time:15 Minutes

Ingredients:

- 1 cup peanut butter (any kind, as long as it's natural and unsweetened)
- 7 oz plain cream cheese
- 3 Tbsp coconut oil
- 1 tsp Stevia/your preferred keto sweetener
- 1 tsp vanilla extract
- ¾ cup ground almonds
- Little pinch of salt

Directions:

1. Line a baking tray with baking paper
2. In a large bowl, mix together all ingredients until thoroughly combined. The mixture might be a little tough to stir at the start, but persevere and it will soften and become easier to combine
3. Roll the mixture into 18 balls and place them onto your prepared tray (like most of these ball/bomb/truffle recipes, this is sticky work!)
4. Place the tray into the fridge for about an hour to allow the bombs to chill and set
5. Store in an airtight container in the fridge

Nutrition Info: Calories: 159;Fat: 14 grams ;Protein: 5 grams ;Total carbs: 5 grams ;Net carbs: 4 grams

Raspberry Cream Fat Bombs

Servings: 13

Cooking Time: 30 Minutes

Ingredients:

- 1 packet raspberry Jello (sugar-free)
- 1 tsp gelatin powder
- ½ cup of boiling water
- ½ cup heavy cream

Directions:

1. Mix Jello and gelatin in boiling water in a medium bowl.
2. Stir in cream slowly and mix it for 1 minute.
3. Divide this mixture into candy molds.
4. Refrigerate them for 30 minutes.
5. Enjoy.

Nutrition Info: Calories 197 Total Fat 19.2 g Saturated Fat 10.1 g Cholesterol 11 mg Sodium 78 mg Total Carbs 7.3 g Sugar 1.2 g Fiber 0.8 g Protein 4.2 g

Almond Butter Cinnamon Bars

Servings: 15

Cooking Time: 0 Minutes

Ingredients:

- ½ Cup of creamed coconut, chopped into chunks
- 1/8 Teaspoon of ground cinnamon
- For the first Icing:
- 1 Tablespoon of non-melted extra virgin coconut oil
- 1 Tablespoon of almond butter
- For the Second Icing:
- 1 Tablespoon of extra virgin almond butter
- ½ Teaspoon of ground cinnamon

Directions:

1. Start by lining a muffin pan with muffin liners.
2. In a large mixing bowl and using both your hands, combine the coconut cream with cinnamon and mix very well.
3. Pat the mixture into the dish; make sure to fill 2 mini loaf sections.
4. Then prepare the first icing by whisking the coconut oil with the almond butter and spread the mixture over the creamed coconut.
5. Put the bars into the freezer for about 6 minutes.

6. In the meantime, prepare the second Icing by whisking the icing almond butter with the cinnamon and drizzle it on top of the bars.
7. Place the bars in the refrigerator for about 30 minutes or for about 8 minutes in the freezer.
8. Cut the frozen batter into bars with a knife.
9. Serve and enjoy your delicious bars!

Nutrition Info: Calories: 160| Fat: 7 g;Carbohydrates: 18g;Fiber: 1g;Protein: 3.2 g

Pina Colada Fat Bombs

Servings: 16

Cooking Time: 1 Hour

Ingredients:

- 2 tsp pineapple essence
- 3 tsp erythritol
- 2 tbsp gelatin
- ½ cup boiling water
- ½ cup coconut cream
- 1 tsp rum extract
- 2 scoops MCT powder

Directions:

1. Mix gelatin with boiling water and erythritol in a bowl.
2. Add pineapple essence and mix well then let it sit for 5 minutes.
3. Stir in coconut cream and rum extract then stir this mixture for 2 minutes.
4. Divide this mixture into silicone molds then refrigerate for 1 hour.
5. Serve.

Nutrition Info: Calories 117 Total Fat 21.2 g Saturated Fat 10.4 g Cholesterol 19.7 mg Sodium 104 mg Total Carbs 7.3 g Sugar 3.4 g Fiber 2 g Protein 8.1 g

Red Velvet Fat Bombs

Servings: 12

Cooking Time: 40 Minutes

Ingredients:
- ¼ cup 90% dark chocolate
- 1/3 cup cream cheese, softened
- ¼ cup butter, softened
- 3 tbsp natvia sweetener
- 1 tsp vanilla extract
- 4 drops red food coloring
- 1/3 cup heavy cream, whipped

Directions:
1. Add chocolate to a heatproof bowl and melt it in a microwave for minute.
2. Whisk cream cheese with butter, natvia, vanilla extract, and food coloring in a bowl using a hand mixer until fluffy.
3. Slowly stir in the melted chocolate while beating the mixture with the hand mixer on medium speed.
4. After 2 minutes of beating, transfer the mixture to a piping bag.
5. Pipe the mixture onto a baking sheet lined with baking paper to make small fat bombs.
6. Place them in the refrigerator for 40 minutes.

7. Garnish the fat bombs with heavy cream.
8. Serve.

Nutrition Info: Calories 213 Total Fat 1g Saturated Fat 15.2 g Cholesterol 13 mg Sodium 52 mg Total Carbs 5.5 g Sugar 1.3 g Fiber 0.5 g Protein 6.1 g

Walnut Brownie Balls

Servings: 15

Cooking Time: 15 Minutes

Ingredients:

- 4 oz 72% cocoa dark chocolate
- 3 Tbsp unsweetened cocoa powder
- 1 cup ground almonds
- 1 cup heavy cream
- 1 tsp Stevia/your preferred keto sweetener
- 1 tsp sea salt
- 1 tsp espresso powder
- 1 cup chopped toasted walnuts

Directions:

1. Place the chocolate into a heatproof bowl over a saucepan of boiling water and stir as it melts, take off the heat and leave to cool
2. Stir together the melted chocolate, cocoa, almonds, cream, sweetener, sea salt, and espresso until completely combined
3. Spread the walnuts onto a plate
4. Roll the chocolate mixture into 15 balls and roll them in the walnuts until the balls are totally coated in walnuts

5. Pop the nut-coated balls onto a plate and allow them to chill in the fridge for at least an hour (you don't need to put them on a paper-lined tray because the nuts will prevent them from sticking)
6. Store the balls in an airtight container in the fridge

Nutrition Info: Calories: 205;Fat: 19 grams ;Protein: 5 grams ;Total carbs: grams ;Net carbs: 5 grams

Raspberry Cheesecake Balls

Servings: 12

Cooking Time: 15 Minutes

Ingredients:

- 1 cup chopped almonds
- 3 Tbsp butter
- 13 oz full fat cream cheese
- ½ cup ground almonds
- 1 tsp Stevia/your preferred keto sweetener
- 1 cup fresh raspberries
- 1 tsp vanilla extract

Directions:

1. Line a baking tray with baking paper and set aside
2. Place the butter into a frying pan and place over a medium-high heat and allow the butter to melt
3. Once the butter has melted, add the chopped almonds to the butter and stir as the almonds toast and become golden brown and fragrant. Take off the heat and set aside
4. In a large bowl, combine the cream cheese, ground almonds, sweetener, raspberries and vanilla extract. Don't worry if the raspberries become mashed up in the cream cheese (they will!)
5. Spread the buttery toasted almonds onto a plate

6. Roll the cream cheese mixture into balls (yes, it will be very sticky but just roll with it!)
7. Roll the balls in the buttery almonds until they're totally coated
8. Place the coated cheesecake balls onto your prepared tray and pop into the fridge to chill and set for an hour or so
9. Store the balls in an airtight container in the fridge

Nutrition Info: Calories: 177;Fat: 16 grams ;Protein: 4 grams ;Total carbs: 5 grams ;Net carbs: 3 grams

Mocha Truffles

Servings: 15

Cooking Time: 10 Minutes

Ingredients:

- 1 cup ground almonds
- 4 Tbsp unsweetened cocoa powder
- 1 tsp Stevia/your preferred keto sweetener
- 3 Tbsp instant espresso powder, dissolved in 2 Tbsp hot water
- 1 cup heavy cream
- 7 oz full fat ricotta cheese

Directions:

1. Line a baking tray with baking paper
2. In a large bowl, thoroughly combine all of the ingredients
3. Roll the mixture into 15 balls and place them onto the lined tray
4. Pop the tray into the fridge to cool and set the truffles for 1 hour
5. Store the truffles in an airtight container in the fridge
6. Serve with a hot coffee!

Nutrition Info: Calories: 124;Fat: 12 grams ;Protein: 3 grams ;Total carbs: 3 grams ;Net carbs: 2 grams

Vanilla Cheesecake Fat Bombs

Servings: 6

Cooking Time: 60 Minutes

Ingredients:

- 9 oz cream cheese, softened
- 2 tsp vanilla extract
- 2 oz erythritol
- 1 cup heavy cream

Directions:

1. In a bowl, mix erythritol, vanilla, and cream cheese with a hand mixer on low speed for two minutes.
2. Slowly add heavy cream to the mixture while beating it continuously until it forms peaks.
3. Divide the mixture into a muffin tray layered with cupcake liners.
4. Place this tray in the refrigerator for 1 hour to set.
5. Enjoy.

Nutrition Info: Calories 173 Total Fat 13 g Saturated Fat 10.1 g Cholesterol 12 mg Sodium mg Total Carbs 7.5 g Sugar 1.2 g Fiber 0.6 g Protein 3.2 g

Salted Macadamia Keto Bombs

Servings: 12

Cooking Time: 0 Minutes

Ingredients:

- 10 Tablespoons of Coconut Oil
- 5 Tablespoons of Unsweetened Cocoa Powder
- 1 Tablespoon of Granulated Stevia
- 3 Tablespoon of coarsely chopped Macadamia Nuts
- 1 Pinch of Coarse Sea Salt to taste

Directions:

1. Melt the coconut oil over the stove.
2. Add the cocoa powder and the granulated Stevia.
3. Mix your ingredients and remove it from the heat.
4. Spoon the mixture into silicone candy moulds until the mould is about ¾ full.
5. Refrigerate the moulds for about minutes.
6. Sprinkle the macadamia nut in each of the silicone moulds and press down; then return the moulds to the refrigerator and let cool for about 30 minutes.
7. Sprinkle macadamia nuts into each well. Press down to distribute the nuts.
8. Once the chocolates are cool and set, remove it from the refrigerator; then let sit at room temperature and sprinkle with coarse salt.

9. Serve and enjoy your delicious macadamia salted balls!

Nutrition Info: Calories: 120| Fat: 13 g;Carbohydrates: 3g;Fiber: 1.3g;Protein: 2.5 g

Peppermint And Chocolate Keto Squares

Servings: 10

Cooking Time: 0 Minutes

Ingredients:

- For the peppermint filling:
- ½ Cup of coconut butter
- 1 Tablespoon of melted coconut oil
- 1 Teaspoon of peppermint extract
- 2 Tablespoons of Stevia
- For the chocolate layer:
- 2 Tablespoons of melted coconut oil
- 4 Oz of 100% dark chocolate

Directions:

1. In a large mixing bowl, combine all together the coconut butter with the melted coconut oil, the peppermint extract and the stevia and mix very well.
2. Pour a small quantity of peppermint mixture into silicone muffin trays to form a layer of about 1/3 inch of thickness.
3. Freeze for about 1 hour; then melt the dark chocolate with the coconut oil and mix again.
4. Remove the firm peppermint filling from the cups.

5. Pour a small quantity of the chocolate mixture into each of the cups in a way that it covers the base; then cover with more chocolate.
6. Repeat the same process with the remaining cups.
7. Let the patties cool for about 2 hours until it becomes solid; then let thaw for about 10 minutes.
8. Serve and enjoy your patties!

Nutrition Info: Calories: 153;Fat: 13 g;Carbohydrates: 3g;Fiber: 2g;Protein: 4 g

Ginger Patties

Servings: 15

Cooking Time: 0 Minutes

Ingredients:

- 1 Cup of coconut butter, softened
- 1 Cup of coconut oil, softened
- ½ Cup of shredded coconut; unsweetened
- 1 Teaspoon of stevia
- 1 Teaspoon of ginger powder

Directions:

1. Mix the softened coconut butter with the coconut oil, the stevia, the shredded coconut and the ginger powder and mix very well until your ingredients are very well dissolved.
2. Pour the batter into the silicon moulds and refrigerate for about 10 minutes.
3. Serve and enjoy your ginger patties.

Nutrition Info: Calories: 123;Fat: 12.7 g;Carbohydrates: 2.;Fiber: 1.2g;Protein: 1.8 g

Coconut Truffles

Servings: 12

Cooking Time: 30 Minutes

Ingredients:

- 2 cups unsweetened coconut thread
- 1 tsp Stevia/your prepared keto sweetener
- 3 egg whites, lightly beaten
- 2 Tbsp coconut flour
- 1 tsp vanilla extract

Directions:

1. Preheat the oven to 350 degrees Fahrenheit and line a baking tray with baking paper
2. Heat a frying pan over a medium heat, do not add any oil to the pan, (it should be dry)
3. Add the coconut thread to the hot pan and stir as it toasts and becomes golden, take off the heat
4. Combine all ingredients in a large bowl
5. Roll the mixture into rough balls and place them onto your prepared tray
6. Place the tray into the oven and bake for about 15 minutes or until the truffles are golden
7. Leave the truffles to cool completely before storing them away in an airtight container

Nutrition Info: Calories: ;Fat: 7 grams ;Protein: 2 grams ;Total carbs: 4 grams ;Net carbs: 2 grams

Keto Ramekin Bread

Servings: 1

Cooking Time: 3 Minutes

Ingredients:

- 1 egg
- 1 tbsp butter
- 3 tbsp almond flour
- ½ tsp baking powder

Directions:

1. Add all the ingredients for keto bread to a small bowl.
2. Pour this batter into a greased ramekin then place in the microwave.
3. Let it cook for 90 seconds on high heat then remove the bread from the ramekin.
4. Cut it in half then add the halves to a greased skillet.
5. Sear the bread in the skillet over medium heat until golden brown on all sides.
6. Enjoy.

Nutrition Info: Calories 1 Total Fat 16.2 g Saturated Fat 9.8 g Cholesterol 100 mg Total Carbs 9.4 g Sugar 0.2 g Fiber 1 g Sodium 42 mg Protein 3.3 g

Apple Cider Bread

Servings: 6

Cooking Time: 20 Minutes

Ingredients:
- 1 egg
- 1/3 cup sour cream
- 1 tbsp + 2 tsp apple cider vinegar
- 2 tbsp water
- 1 cup almond flour
- 5 tbsp golden flaxseed meal
- 3 tbsp coconut flour
- 1/3 cup whey protein isolate
- 3 ½ tsp baking powder
- 1 tsp xanthan gum
- ½ tsp kosher salt
- 8 tbsp butter, melted

Directions:
1. Preheat your oven to 350 degrees F.
2. Layer a baking tray with wax paper and set it aside.
3. Beat eggs with apple cider vinegar, water, and sour cream in a medium bowl.
4. Grind flaxseed meal with almond flour, whey protein, coconut flour, salt, baking powder, and xanthan gum in a food processor.

5. Add butter and egg mixture and blend again until smooth.
6. Spread the batter in the baking tray.
7. Brush the top with melted butter then bake for 20 minutes.
8. Let them cool for 10 minutes.
9. Slice and serve.

Nutrition Info: Calories 214 Total Fat 19 g Saturated Fat 5.8 g Cholesterol 15 mg Sodium 123 mg Total Carbs 6.5 g Sugar 1.9 g Fiber 2.1 g Protein 6.5 g

Keto Cream Cheese Bread

Servings: 6

Cooking Time: 30 Minutes

Ingredients:

- 8 large eggs
- 8 oz full-fat cream cheese
- ½ cup unsalted butter
- 1 ½ cups coconut flour
- ½ cup full-fat sour cream
- 4 tsp baking powder
- 1 tsp sea salt
- 1 tbsp Swerve
- 2 tbsp sesame seeds

Directions:

1. Preheat your oven to 350 degrees F.
2. Grease a 10-inch loaf pan with butter liberally.
3. Whisk baking powder, sweetener, salt, and coconut flour together in a medium-size bowl.
4. Beat cream cheese with butter in a bowl until fluffy using a hand mixer.
5. Add eggs one by one while beating the mixture.
6. Add flour mixture and combine until smooth.
7. Fold in the sour cream and mix well until incorporated.

8. Spread this dough into the prepared pan.
9. Bake it for 30 minutes until golden brown.
10. Enjoy.

Nutrition Info: Calories 282 Total Fat 25.1 g Saturated Fat 8.8 g Cholesterol 100 mg Sodium mg Total Carbs 9.4 g Sugar 0.7 g Fiber 3.2 g Protein 8 g

Low Carb Flax Bread

Servings: 8

Cooking Time: 20 Minutes

Ingredients:

- ½ cup ground flaxseeds
- ½ cup psyllium husk powder
- 1 tbsp baking powder
- 1 ½ cups soy protein isolate
- ¼ cup granulated stevia
- 2 tsp salt
- 7 large egg whites
- 1 large whole egg
- 3 tbsp butter
- ¾ cup of water

Directions:

1. Preheat your oven to 350 degrees F.
2. Whisk baking powder, ground flaxseed, psyllium husk, stevia, protein, and salt in a bowl.
3. Beat egg with butter, water, and egg whites in a separate bowl.
4. Mix these two mixtures together until smooth.
5. Grease a loaf pan with cooking oil then spread the batter in it.
6. Bake it for 20 minutes until it is done.

7. Enjoy.

Nutrition Info: Calories 207 Total Fat 19 g Saturated Fat 14 g Cholesterol 111 mg Sodium 122 mg Total Carbs 7 g Sugar 1 g Fiber 3 g Protein 6 g

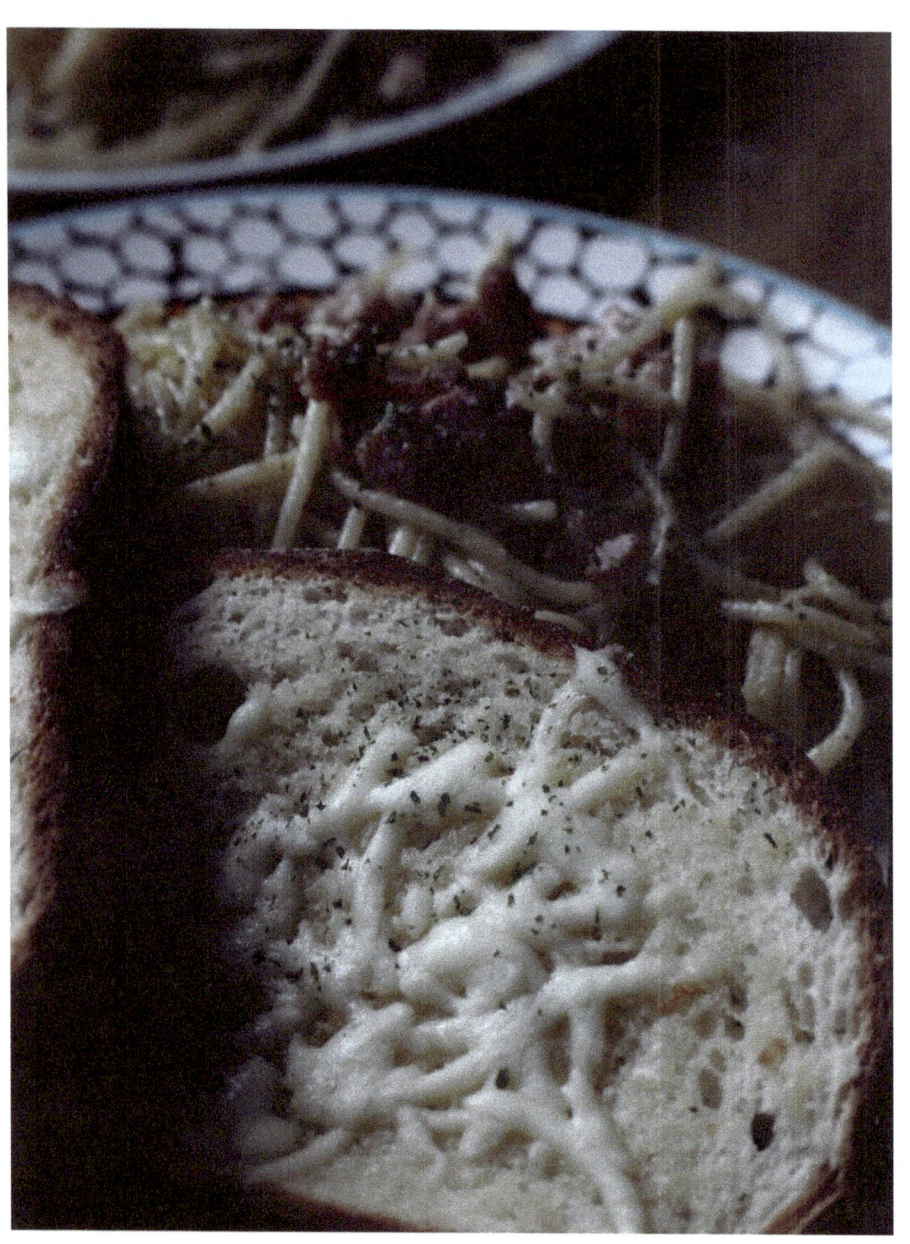

Gluten-free Garlic Bread

Servings: 4-5

Cooking Time: 40 Minutes

Ingredients:

- 2 egg whites
- 1 and ¼ cups of boiling water
- 2 teaspoons of apple cider vinegar
- 1 Teaspoon of sea salt
- 2 Teaspoons of baking powder
- 5 Tbsps of ground Psyllium husk powder
- 1 and ¼ cups of almond flour
- For the Garlic butter: ½ Teaspoon of salt + 1 Minced garlic clove + 4 Oz of butter + 2 Tbsp of finely chopped parsley

Directions:

1. Preheat your oven to around 360 F and then combine your dry ingredients into a deep and large mixing bowl.
2. Pour the boiling water; then add the egg whites and the vinegar to the bowl and keep whisking for around 1 minute, but make sure to not over mix.
3. With moist hands, form around 10 pieces.
4. Roll the 10 pieces into buns and then place them over a baking sheet.

5. Bake your buns for around 40 minutes in the oven. Meanwhile, prepare the garlic butter by mixing its ingredients and then refrigerate it.
6. Once your buns are ready, set it aside to cool for around 10 minutes.
7. Cut the buns into halves and then spread the butter on every half.
8. Raise the heat to around 425 F and then bake it for about 15 minutes.
9. Serve and enjoy!

Nutrition Info: Calories: 180;Fat: 9 g;Carbohydrates: 12g;Fiber: 1 g;Protein: 5 g

Zucchini Bread With Walnuts

Servings: 8

Cooking Time: 70 Minutes

Ingredients:

- 3 large eggs
- ½ cup olive oil
- 1 tsp vanilla extract
- 2 ½ cups almond flour
- 1 ½ cups erythritol
- ½ tsp salt
- 1 ½ tsp baking powder
- ½ tsp nutmeg
- 1 tsp ground cinnamon
- ¼ tsp ground ginger
- 1 cup grated zucchini
- ½ cup chopped walnuts

Directions:

1. Preheat your oven to 350 degrees F.
2. Beat eggs with vanilla extract and oil in a mixer.
3. Whisk almond flour with baking powder, salt, erythritol, ginger, cinnamon, and nutmeg in a separate bowl.
4. Stir in egg mixture and mix well until incorporated.

5. Place zucchini in cheesecloth and squeeze the excess water out of it.
6. Add this zucchini to the egg and flour mixture then mix well.
7. Grease a 9x5-inch loaf pan with cooking oil and spread the batter in the pan.
8. Sprinkle chopped walnuts on top then bake for 70 minutes at 350 degrees F.
9. Slice and serve.

Nutrition Info: Calories 201 Total Fat 12.2 g Saturated Fat 2.4 g Cholesterol 1mg Sodium 276 mg Total Carbs 4.3 g Fiber 0.9 g Sugar 1.4 g Protein 8.8 g

Cheesy Keto Garlic Bread

Servings: 6

Cooking Time: 15 Minutes

Ingredients:

- 1¾ cups grated cheese mozzarella
- ¾ cups almond flour
- 2 tbsp cream cheese, full fat
- 1 tsp baking powder
- Pinch salt, to taste
- 1 medium egg
- Glaze:
- 1 tbsp garlic, crushed
- 1 tbsp parsley, fresh or dried
- 2 tbsp butter, melted

Directions:

1. Add everything except the egg to a microwave-safe bowl.
2. Heat this mixture for 1 minute in the microwave on High.
3. Stir well then heat again for seconds in the microwave.
4. Whisk in egg and stir well to form the dough.
5. Spread this dough in a greased loaf pan and set aside.
6. Prepare the glaze by mixing butter with garlic.
7. Brush this mixture liberally over the bread.

8. Bake for 15 minutes at 425 degrees F until golden.
9. Enjoy.

Nutrition Info: Calories 158 Total Fat 15.2 g Saturated Fat 5.2 g Cholesterol 269 mg Sodium 178 mg Total Carbs 7.4 g Sugar 1.1 g Fiber 3.5 g Protein 5.5 g

Morning Hamburger Loaves

Servings: 1

Cooking Time: 1.5 Minutes

Ingredients:

- 1 large egg
- 1 tbsp almond flour
- 1 tbsp psyllium husk powder
- ¼ tsp baking powder
- ¼ tsp cream of tartar
- 1 tbsp chicken broth
- 1 tbsp melted butter

Directions:

1. Crack an egg in a wide microwave-safe mug.
2. Pour melted butter over the egg and let it sit for 1 minute.
3. Stir in almond flour, baking powder, chicken broth, cream of tartar, and husk powder.
4. Mix well to form a smooth batter then place the mug in the microwave.
5. Bake it for 7seconds in the microwave on High.
6. Slice and serve.

Nutrition Info: Calories 248 Total Fat 19.3 g Saturated Fat 4.8 g Cholesterol 32 mg Sodium 59mg Total Carbs 3.1 g Fiber 0.6 g Sugar 1.9 g Protein 7.9 g

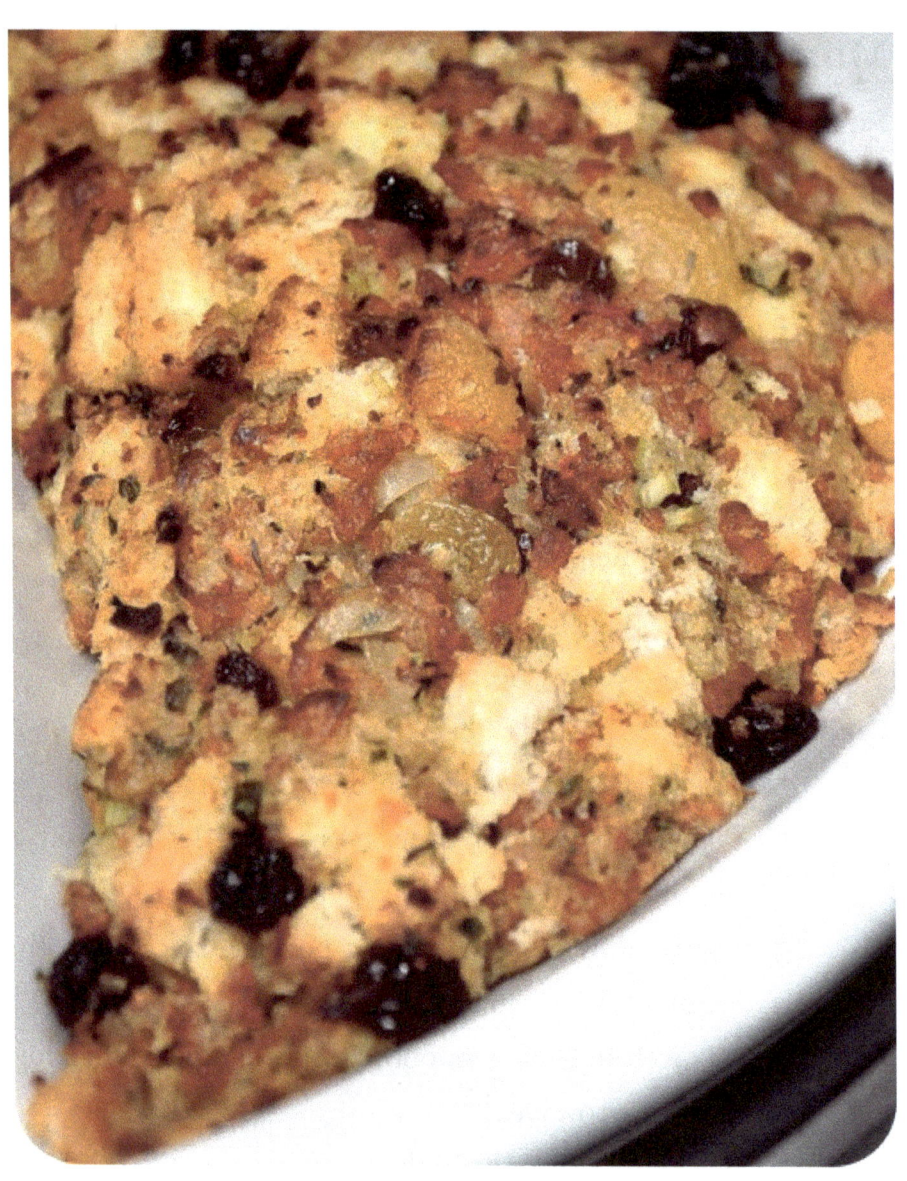

Savory Sage Bread

Servings: 12

Cooking Time: 35 Minutes

Ingredients:

- 2 ½ cups almond flour
- ¼ cup coconut flour
- ½ cup butter
- 8 oz cream cheese
- 8 whole eggs
- 1 tsp rosemary
- 1 tsp sage
- 2 tbsp parsley
- 1 ½ tsp baking powder

Directions:

1. Beat half cup butter and 8 oz cream cheese in a medium-size bowl with a hand mixer until smooth.
2. Stir in rosemary, parsley, and sage then mix well.
3. Whisk in eggs while beating until mixture is smooth.
4. Add baking powder along with flours and mix well until it forms a thick batter.
5. Grease three small loaf pans and divide the batter into these pans.
6. Place them in the oven and bake the batter for 35 minutes at 350 degrees F.

7. Serve once cooled.

Nutrition Info: Calories 255 Total Fat 23.4 g Saturated Fat 11.7 g Cholesterol 135 mg Sodium 112 mg Total Carbs 2.5 g Sugar 12.5 g Fiber 1 g Protein 7.9 g

Cinnamon Bread

Servings: 6

Cooking Time: 45 Minutes

Ingredients:

- 1 and ½ cups of almond flour
- ¾ Teaspoon of baking soda
- ½ Teaspoon of baking powder
- ¼ Teaspoon of salt
- 1 Teaspoon of cinnamon
- ½ Teaspoon of ground all spice
- 4Tbsp of butter
- 2 Large organic eggs
- 1 Cup of avocado puree
- ½ Cup of heavy cream
- ½ Tbsp of grated lemon zest

Directions:

1. Preheat your oven to 340 F and line a loaf pan with parchment paper; then set it aside.
2. In a deep bowl, combine all together the baking powder, the salt, the lemon zest, the all spice and the cinnamon and mix very well.
3. Pour the butter in a bowl and with a hand mixer beat it until it becomes soft and very smooth.

4. Add in the eggs and the avocado puree then carry on mixing the ingredients.
5. Add your dry mixture and the heavy cream into your batter and mix it very well until it is very well combined.
6. Transfer your batter to your already prepared loaf pan then bake it for around 45 minutes.
7. After around 45 minutes, poke the bread with the knife.
8. Remove your bread from the oven and set it aside to cool on a rack.
9. Set the bread aside to cool down and after that, slice it.
10. Serve and enjoy it!

Nutrition Info: Calories: 173;Fat: 15 g;Carbohydrates: 2g;Fiber: 2 g;Protein: 6 g

Cloud Bread

Servings: 4

Cooking Time: 25 Minutes

Ingredients:

- 3 eggs
- 3 tbsp coconut cream
- ½ tsp baking powder
- 1 Pinch sea salt
- 1 pinch black pepper
- 1 pinch dried rosemary

Directions:

1. Preheat your oven to 325 degrees F. Layer a baking sheet with wax paper.
2. Separate the egg yolks from the whites then add the yolks to a bowl with the coconut cream.
3. Beat well with a hand mixer until fluffy.
4. Whisk egg whites with baking powder in a separate bowl using the hand mixer.
5. Beat it until thick and foamy.
6. Add the egg yolk mixture to the whites and mix well.
7. Drop the batter onto the baking sheet spoon by spoon to get 4-inch separate circles.
8. Bake them for 25 minutes in the oven.
9. Enjoy.

Nutrition Info: Calories 233 Total Fat 20.2 g Saturated Fat 4.4 g Cholesterol 120 mg Sodium 76 mg Total Carbs 3.5 g Fiber 0.9 g Sugar 1.4 g Protein 1.9 g

Almond Flour Bread With Olive

Servings: 5

Cooking Time: 45 Minutes

Ingredients:

- 2 Cups of golden flaxseed flour
- 5 Beaten egg whites
- 2 Yolks of egg
- 4 tbsps of olive oil
- 1 tbsp of baking powder
- 2 tbsps of apple cider vinegar
- 2 tbsps of Psyllium husk powder
- ½ Teaspoon of salt
- 6 Finely chopped sundried tomatoes
- ½ Cup of chopped black olives
- 1 Cup of feta cheese
- 1 Tbsp of dried oregano
- 1 Tbsp of dried thyme
- ½ Cup of boiling water

Directions:

1. Preheat your oven to around 350 F.
2. Grease a small bread pan and line it with a parchment paper.
3. Combine the flaxseed, the baking powder and the Psyllium in a deep bowl.

4. Add the oil and the eggs and mix very well until you notice the mixture becoming like breadcrumbs.
5. Pour in the cider vinegar and combine the mixture; then add boiling water and keep stirring until your mixture starts to resemble dough.
6. Add the olives, the feta cheese and the dried tomato.
7. Pour your batter in the greased loaf pan.
8. Bake the bread loaf for about 45 minutes.
9. Slice the bread loaf; then serve and enjoy it!

Nutrition Info: Calories: 189;Fat: 14 g;Carbohydrates: 8g;Fiber: 1.1g;Protein: 9 g

Low Carb Blueberry Bread

Servings: 12

Cooking Time: 45 Minutes

Ingredients:

- ½ cup almond butter
- ¼ cup butter
- ½ cup almond flour
- ½ tsp salt
- 2 tsp baking powder
- ½ cup almond milk, unsweetened
- 5 eggs, beaten
- ½ cup blueberries

Directions:

1. Preheat your oven to 350 degrees F.
2. Melt the butter in a bowl in the microwave then mix well.
3. Whisk almond butter with salt, baking powder, and almond flour in a suitable bowl.
4. Stir in almond milk and egg while beating the mixture.
5. Fold in berries and mix gently.
6. Layer a loaf pan with wax paper and grease it lightly with cooking oil.
7. Pour the blueberry batter into the loaf pan.
8. Bake for 45 minutes.

9. Allow it to cool on a wire rack for 30 minutes.
10. Slice and serve.

Nutrition Info: Calories 107 Total Fat 9.3 g Saturated Fat 4.8 g Cholesterol 77 mg Sodium 135 mg Total Carbs 2.6 g Fiber 0.8 g Sugar 9.9 g Protein 3.9 g

Jalapeno Cornbread Loaves

Servings: 8

Cooking Time: 22 Minutes

Ingredients:

- Dry Ingredients
- 1 ½ cups almond flour
- ½ cup golden flaxseed meal
- 2 tsp baking powder
- 1 tsp salt
- Wet Ingredients
- ½ cup sour cream, full fat
- 4 tbsp butter, melted
- 4 large eggs
- 10 drops liquid stevia
- 1 tsp Amoretti sweet corn extract
- Add-Ins
- ½ cup sharp cheddar cheese, grated
- 2 fresh jalapenos, seeded and ribs removed
- Sliced jalapenos, for topping

Directions:

1. Preheat your oven to 375 degrees F.
2. Grease a mini loaf pan with cooking oil or butter.
3. Mix almond flour, salt, baking powder, and flaxseed meal in a bowl.

4. Whisk wet ingredients in a separate bowl then stir in the dry mixture.
5. After mixing it well, fold in the chopped pepper and cheddar cheese.
6. Spread this batter evenly in the loaf pan and place additional sliced pepper rings on top.
7. Bake the loaf for 22 minutes until golden brown.
8. Slice and serve.

Nutrition Info: Calories 301 Total Fat 26.3 g Saturated Fat 14.8 g Cholesterol 322 mg Sodium 5 mg Total Carbs 2.6 g Fiber 0.6 g Sugar 1.9 g Protein 12 g

Walnut Bread

Servings: 5-6

Cooking Time: 35 Minutes

Ingredients:

- ½ Tbsp of butter
- ¼ Cup of chopped onion
- 4 Tbsps of chopped walnuts
- ¾ Cup of almond flour
- 4 Tbsps of coconut flour
- ½ teaspoon of baking soda
- ¼ Teaspoon of salt
- ¼ Teaspoon of nutmeg
- 2 Large organic eggs
- 4 Tbsps of beef broth

Directions:

1. Start by preheating your oven to around 350 F.
2. Line a loaf tray with a parchment paper and set it aside. Meanwhile, melt the butter into a medium saucepan on a medium heat.
3. Add the onion and the walnuts to your saucepan.
4. Sauté the ingredients for around 2 to 3 minutes.
5. In a large bowl, combine the almond flour with the coconut flour, the baking soda, the salt, and the nutmeg and whisk very well.

6. Add the sautéed onion and the walnuts into your dry mixture with the eggs and the beef broth.
7. Whisk the mixture until it is perfectly combined.
8. Transfer your mixture into the already prepared loaf tray and then spread it evenly.
9. Bake the loaf of bread for around 35 minutes or insert a tooth pick to check if it is done.
10. Turn off the heat and remove your loaf from the oven and set it aside for minutes.
11. Slice the bread; then serve and enjoy!

Nutrition Info: Calories: 90;Fat: 6.8 g;Carbohydrates 3.8g;Fiber: 0.52 g;Protein: 5.3 g

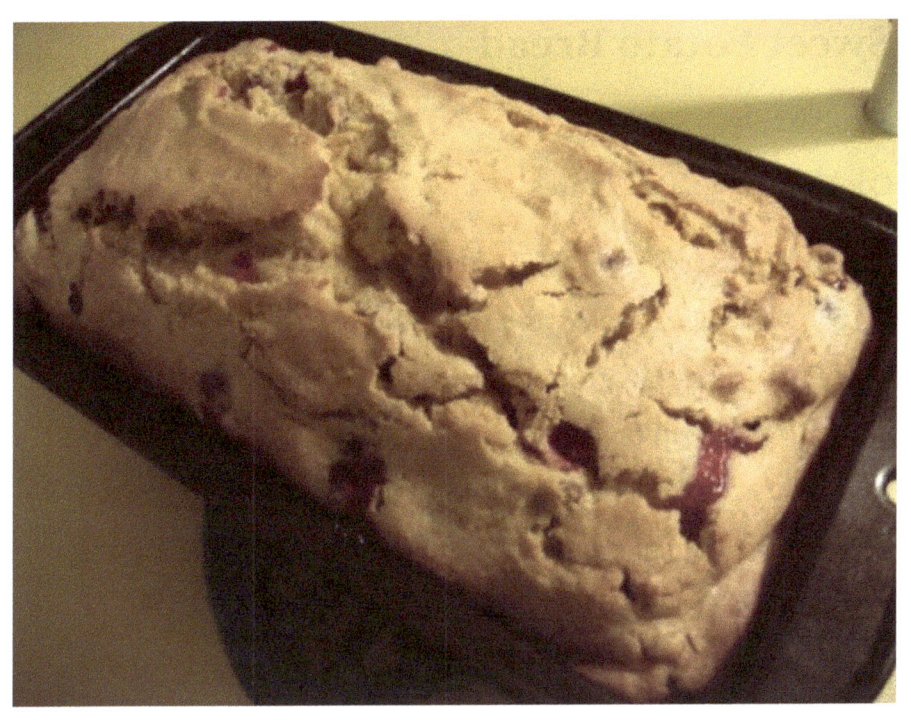

Sweet Potato Bread

Servings: 5

Cooking Time: 45 Minutes

Ingredients:

- 1 large peeled and diced sweet potato
- 1 Tbsp of ground flaxseeds
- 3 Tbsp of water
- 2 and ½ cups of almond flour
- 1 Teaspoon of dried thyme
- 1 Teaspoon of fresh chopped rosemary
- ½ Teaspoon of sea salt
- 2 Tbsp of extra-virgin olive oil

Directions:

1. Preheat your oven to around 350 F.
2. Steam your sweet potatoes into a steamer basket in an instant pot or boil steam it in a steamer basket above the stove on top of boiling water for around 6 to 9 minutes.
3. Mix the flax seeds with water in a deep bowl and set it aside for around 10 minutes.
4. Mix again very well and mash the cooked potatoes with a potato masher or with a fork.

5. Add the rest of the ingredients and then add the rest of the ingredients and mix all the ingredients together very well.
6. Form the dough from your mixture and transfer your dough to a lined parchment and roll the dough with a rolling pin into around ½ inch of thickness.
7. Bake the dough for about 40 to 45 minutes.
8. Once the bread becomes brown, remove it from the oven and set it aside to cool down for around 20 minutes.
9. Cut the bread into rectangles.
10. Serve and enjoy!

Nutrition Info: Calories: 100;Fat: 3 g;Carbohydrates: ;Fiber: 1 g;Protein: 4.9 g

Coconut Bread

Servings: 10

Cooking Time: 50 Minutes

Ingredients:

- ½ cup coconut flour
- ¼ tsp salt
- ¼ tsp baking soda
- 6 eggs
- ¼ cup coconut oil, melted
- ¼ unsweetened almond milk

Directions:

1. Preheat your oven to 350 degrees F. Layer an 8x4-inch loaf pan with wax paper.
2. Mix coconut flour with salt and baking soda in a suitable bowl.
3. Whisk eggs with oil and milk in a separate bowl.
4. Stir coconut flour mixture into the egg mixture and combine until smooth.
5. Spread this bread batter in the loaf pan.
6. Bake it for 50 minutes until it is done.
7. Allow it to cool then slice and enjoy.

Nutrition Info: Calories 192 Total Fat 11.g Saturated Fat 3.9 g Cholesterol 135 mg Sodium 187 mg Total Carbs 4.1 g Fiber 0.1g Sugar 2.1 g Protein 5.9 g

Flax Seed Bread

Servings: 6

Cooking Time: 30 Minutes

Ingredients:

- 1 Teaspoon of salt
- 1/3 Cup of olive oil
- 2 Cups of flax seed meal
- ½ Cup of water
- 1 Tbsp of baking powder
- 2 Tbsp of maple syrup
- 4 to 5 beaten pasteurised eggs

Directions:

1. Preheat the oven to around 350 F.
2. Line a 10*15 inch baking tray with parchment paper.
3. Whisk together your dry ingredients then add them to the wet ingredients to your dry ingredients and combine the mixture very well.
4. Set the batter aside for around 3 minutes until it thickens up.
5. Pour your batter into your already prepared tray and spread it into the bottom; but make sure to keep it away from sides of the pan.
6. Spread the batter into the shape of a rectangle for about 1 inch or 2 from the end of the pan.

7. Place the baking pan in the oven and bake it for around 30 minutes.
8. Once the bread gets brown, remove it from the oven and set it aside to cool down for around 5 minutes.
9. Slice the bread then serve and enjoy it!

Nutrition Info: Calories: 187;Fat: 11 g;Carbohydrates: 7g;Fiber: 4g;Protein: 8 g

Keto Breadsticks

Servings: 6

Cooking Time: 15 Minutes

Ingredients:

- Bread Stick Base
- 2 cups mozzarella cheese, shredded
- ¾ cup almond flour
- 1 tbsp psyllium husk powder
- 3 tbsp cream cheese
- 1 large egg
- 1 tsp baking powder
- Italian Spice Mix
- 2 tbsp Italian seasoning
- 1 tsp salt
- 1 tsp pepper
- Extra Cheese Topping
- 1 tsp garlic powder
- 1 tsp onion powder
- 3 oz cheddar cheese
- ¼ cup parmesan cheese

Directions:

1. Preheat your oven to 400 degrees F.
2. Whisk egg with cream cheese in a bowl and set it aside.

3. Mix almond flour, baking powder, and psyllium husk in a separate bowl.
4. Heat mozzarella cheese in a large bowl in the microwave for 20 seconds.
5. Mix well then stir in cream cheese, egg, and dry mixture.
6. Continue mixing then knead this dough on your work surface.
7. Spread this dough into a flat thick sheet then place it on a baking sheet.
8. Mix everything for the Italian spice mix and sprinkle it over the dough.
9. Mix everything for the cheese topping and spread that over the dough.
10. Bake the dough for 15 minutes until crispy.
11. Slice into long sticks.
12. Serve with a cream cheese dip or your favourite spread.
13. Enjoy.

Nutrition Info: Calories 216 Total Fat 20.9 g Saturated Fat 8.1 g Cholesterol 241 mg Total Carbs 8.3 g Sugar 1.8 g Fiber 3.8 g Sodium 8 mg Protein 6.4 g

Cranberry Bread

Servings: 12

Cooking Time: 1 Hour & 15 Minutes

Ingredients:

- 2 cups almond flour
- ½ cup powdered erythritol
- ½ tsp stevia powder
- 1 ½ tsp baking powder
- ½ tsp baking soda
- 1 tsp salt
- 4 tbsp unsalted butter, melted
- 1 tsp blackstrap molasses
- 4 large eggs
- ½ cup coconut milk
- 1 12-oz bag cranberries

Directions:

1. Preheat your oven to 350 degrees F. Grease a 9x5-inch loaf pan with cooking oil.
2. Mix flour with baking powder, baking soda, stevia, salt, and erythritol in a large bowl.
3. Whisk eggs with molasses, coconut milk, and butter in a separate bowl.
4. Stir in sweet flour mixture and combine until smooth.
5. Fold in the cranberries and mix gently.

6. Spread this berry batter in a loaf pan then bake for 1 hour and 15 minutes.
7. Check the bread after 1 hour by inserting a toothpick. Bake more if toothpick doesn't come out clean.
8. Place it on a wire rack to cool down.
9. Slice and serve.

Nutrition Info: Calories 172 Total Fat 7 g Saturated Fat 7.4 g Cholesterol 62 mg Sodium 121 mg Total Carbs 4.9 g Fiber 0.6 g Sugar 17.3 g Protein 4 g

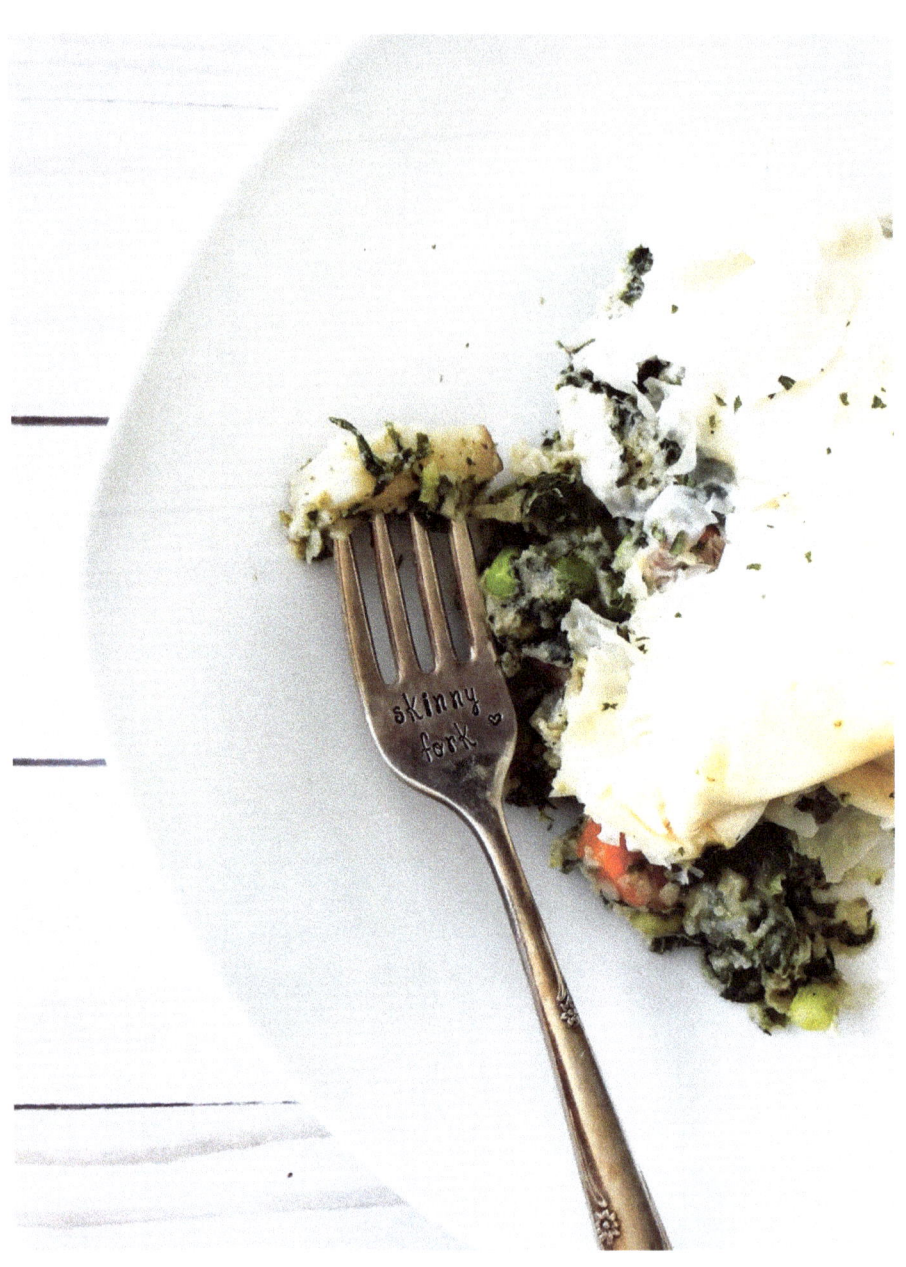

www.ingramcontent.com/pod-product-compliance
Lightning Source LLC
Chambersburg PA
CBHW071107030426
42336CB00013BA/1991